YOGA
A PATH TO AWARENESS

YOGA
A PATH TO AWARENESS

COLLECTED ESSAYS

SWAMI SIVANANDA RADHA

TIMELESS
2016

timeless books
www.timeless.org

in Canada:
P.O. Box 9, Kootenay Bay, BC, VOB 1X0
contact@timeless.org
(800) 661-8711

in the US:
P.O. Box 3543, Spokane, WA, 99220-3543
info@timeless.org
(800) 251-9273

Design by Todd Stewart
Cover and author photo courtesy of Yasodharā Ashram
Essays originally published in *Ascent* magazine, 1999-2009

Library and Archives Canada Cataloguing in Publication

Radha, Swami Sivananda, 1911–1995, author
Yoga : A path to awareness : collected essays / Swami Sivananda Radha.

ISBN 978-1-932018-60-8 (paperback)

1. Yoga. 2. Self-actualization (Psychology). I. Title.

B132.Y6R23 2016 204'.36 C2016-904548-X

Printed in Canada
Interior: FSC® certified 100% post-consumer-waste recycled acid-free paper
Cover: FSC® certified 10% post-consumer-waste recycled paper

Environmental Benefits Statement

By using paper made with post-consumer recycled content, the following resources have been saved.

trees	water	energy	solid waste	greenhouse gases
8	14,258	4	115	315
fully grown	litres	million BTU	kilograms	kilograms

Environmental impact estimates were made using the Environmental Paper Network Calculator. For more information visit http://calculator.environmentalpaper.org

FSC www.fsc.org MIX Paper from responsible sources FSC® C014956

zero 100% carbon neutral by Hemlock Printers www.hemlock.com/zero

Also by Swami Sivananda Radha

Radha: Diary of a Woman's Search
Hatha Yoga: The Hidden Language
In the Company of the Wise: A Disciple's Path
Kundalini Yoga for the West
The Divine Light Invocation
On Sanyas: The Yoga of Renunciation
Light and Vibration
The Yoga of Healing
Mantras: Words of Power
When You First Called Me Radha: Poems
The Devi of Speech: The Goddess in Kundalini Yoga
The Rose Ceremony
Realities of the Dreaming Mind
Time to be Holy: Collected Satsang Talks

Table of Contents

Introduction

SHE was born to a wealthy Berlin family in 1911, an only child in a marriage that ended in early divorce. Sent to a (boys!) boarding school as a young girl, she became the first woman to graduate from a school of advertising, design and photography. A published writer of short stories and a professional interpretive dancer, she married a baron who was deeply in love with her but was soon executed in a Nazi concentration camp for helping Jews escape. She married again. He was a composer and musician – he played, she danced. He died in her arms just a few years later. She became a refugee, fleeing the Russians at the end of World War II and emigrating to England to work as a maid, and then to Canada to work as a secretary.

It is probably not the background that comes to mind when you think of *swami, yogi, guru*. But that was indeed Swami Radha's past – a life filled with challenges and dramas, love and despair. She was 44 when she left Montréal for India in 1955. As a new immigrant to Canada, she had only recently upgraded to a decent apartment and had some promising leads to perform dance.

But her driving desire to know the purpose of her life was a force she could not deny. Her transformative journey to Sivananda Ashram in Rishikesh, India is documented in her book, *Radha: Diary of a Woman's Search*. It is an honest account that includes her doubts and criticism, and her penchant for asking questions that led Gurudev Sivananda to say, "She is a ball of fire – she wants to know!"

When Swami Sivananda sent her back from India to Canada in 1956 as a new swami, she was told to wear her orange robes and to live on faith, not working for money but accepting what came to her. Swami Sivananda didn't understand that in Canada she was more likely to be arrested than worshipped for chanting, dancing and singing holy songs in parks. There was not a tradition of supporting renunciates in North America, but rather of rejecting those who couldn't support themselves.

Swami Radha surrendered to her commitment and found that she was indeed given what she needed in unexpected ways. She also understood that she had to adapt the teachings, which were shaped by the Eastern culture, to the Western mind. She built on her experience and her practices. She passed on what she knew.

As she says in this book:

> *The emphasis in my teaching is on self-examination and self-inquiry. I use familiar Western terms, but in a kind of Eastern psychology that explores each person's*

individual symbolism and use of metaphor, and teaches the practice of awareness.

She started an ashram, as Swami Sivananda had requested, first in Burnaby, BC, a suburb of Vancouver. Then she founded Yasodhara Ashram in its current location at Kootenay Bay, in the mountains of southeast British Columbia – a refuge where she felt people could let go of the busyness of their city lives and think deeply about their direction and purpose.

Slowly others gathered around to support the work, which was initially the Karma Yoga of clearing land for gardens, building humble accommodations and meditation spaces, and learning to live and work together as a small community. Swami Radha traveled throughout Canada and the United States, taught at transpersonal institutes and lectured at conferences. She helped establish the beginnings of the Eastern spirituality movement of North America in the 1960s and 70s.

She wrote books, including the classic yoga texts, *Kundalini Yoga for the West* and *Hatha Yoga: the Hidden Language*. She started small centres throughout North America led by dedicated students. She initiated others into the lineage through *mantra*, *brahmacharya* and *sanyas*. Until her passing in 1995, she continued to write, to support and challenge her disciples, and to establish a lineage led by women.

Early on, Swami Radha formed her own publishing company, Timeless Books, so her writing would not be compromised in any way for higher sales. There is indeed a timeless quality to her work.

For example, this passage, written several decades ago, applies more than ever today:

> *Life these days has become very complex. There is such an enormous input of information that our heads begin to whirl – we don't know what to do with it all. So first we need to take a good look at ourselves and ask, "How do I experience life?"*

I was Swami Radha's editor for seven years, and am happy to see this collection of her essays, originally published in *Ascent* magazine, gathered here.

What I so appreciate about Swami Radha's life and work is her integrity, how her life reflected what she taught. As I reviewed this collection I was touched by the power of her words, and how they resonated for me personally, and how they reflected the way she herself lived. Her advice to others was based on her own deep exploration, experimentation, and understanding of what it takes to walk the spiritual path. She understood the stages, the obstacles, the desires and fantasies, the need to discern. She lived a life of loving the Divine and not fooling herself.

Her only concern was "to help regardless of any return or recognition." She lived a life of continuous learning and encouraged others to do the same. She not only bridged the worlds of East and West, but of practicality and spirituality, bringing spiritual concepts down to earth. "Face the facts and aim for Higher Consciousness," she says.

She is one who lived her words. And so her words live on.

With gratitude,
Swami Lalitananda
President, Yasodhara Ashram
March 2016

1 LIBERATION: THE PATH OF YOGA

1 Liberation

YOGA IS A PATH of liberation, and liberation has to begin in the here and now of our daily lives. We have to liberate ourselves from our own self-made prisons. These are prisons of attachments, concepts and habits, and the compelling forces of mechanical reactions and untested beliefs.

Where are you imprisoned? You may feel there are areas, such as your work situation, where you didn't create the prison – the eight-hour workday five days a week, the tough boss, the lack of recognition, the low salary, or whatever the situation is. But do you have to stay in that prison? No. Sometimes it is your own lack of courage that keeps you prisoner. Many people feel comfortable in the security they've created and yet are angry with themselves for needing such security because it prevents them from trying something new. They also may have spent whatever they've earned, leaving no money to pay for additional training or education. Or they may have become lazy in their thinking and blame life or destiny for circumstances that they themselves have created.

Always remember you are the doer, and you can undo. You have the power of choice, which is often not recognized. Take responsibility for the choices you have made in your life – for your job, your education, your marriage partner, your desire for spiritual life. The power of choice is yours. You even have the power to make changes if you discover that your original choices did not meet your expectations.

How can new decisions be made? First, get all of the facts together about what you want to do. Generate options. Pay attention to your emotional responses to the various possibilities because where your joy is the greatest, there you will succeed – even if you think you have little to offer or you have little capital to enter into any new business or professional venture.

We learn by trial and error, and all great things in life have been achieved by trial and error. So we have to try. Your past mistakes are also not important. We have all made our mistakes. I have made my own, therefore I would never be in a position to judge others. But what is it you want to do now? Where do you want to go from here? If you step onto the royal highway towards a spiritual goal – which you have to define and lay out for yourself because it is your path and it is your life – then you have to take responsibility for what you do. And you must try your very best not to repeat past mistakes, even if you occasionally slip. If you do slip, forgive yourself but carry on. It is important to make a clear decision of will. If you can turn your stubbornness into properly directed willpower, you will be successful in reaching your spiritual goal because perseverance is needed.

Spiritual liberation is not possible unless you lay a good, solid foundation in your daily life – building character and taking responsibility for yourself. Daydreaming will not lead to liberation. You can't just think about it. You have to take action. You have to take your life very firmly into your own hands.

How can we become aware? Where shall we begin? Again, we want to be practical. Look into your habits. Look into those mechanical reactions, things that you do over and over again with little change. Keep a daily diary in which you write your reflections on your daily actions and become aware of how mechanical, almost robotic you can be. Observe how difficult it is to drop your grudges and negative thinking. Not only do we have to undo the selfishness from this life, but we also have an accumulation of karma from many lives. Life is like the battleground of the Bhagavad Gita. Wherever you are, you battle your own selfishness, you battle your own many personality aspects and you battle your illusions.

As you work on yourself ask, Have I changed? What have I accomplished in my attempts towards self-mastery? When you begin to clearly see your self-made prisons and limitations, then you will slowly start to understand what the word "liberation" means. Usually we have a theoretical understanding. We intellectualize very cleverly about all these things but haven't necessarily accomplished anything.

So we have to be clear. Tell yourself the truth about yourself – that you are just starting out on the path. The liberation that you are aiming for will come by degrees, and so will meditation. Without the ability to concentrate, there is very little possibility of results. Making the mind a blank is not meditation. Triggering yourself into a state of trance is not meditation. Meditation comes when the mind is calm, and that calmness comes only when you stop scheming to fulfill selfish desires.

There is no sudden miracle where all of your negative characteristics just drop away. It is a Western misconception that if you meditate eight hours a day like the yogis in India all your shortcomings will disappear. They won't. We have to work on ourselves. God will not do it for us. No true teacher will do it for you. You must take responsibility for yourself. You are the doer of the wrong actions in the past, so you are also the one who can undo them.

It is my prayer that you all have the courage, the determination and the persistence to undo your self-made prisons. Awareness is the key. Recognize the key. Find the door, put the key in the lock and open the door.

Courageously step into that new freedom.

2 The Potential of Selflessness

SWAMI SIVANANDA, in his farewell address to me, said, "Don't be concerned about *samadhi* or realization. Selfless service will make you Divine."

What could he mean?

"Self-less." Less the self. When the physical or mental pain of another person strikes a chord of compassion within, when our only concern is to help regardless of any return or recognition, then we have truly helped selflessly. Selflessness is an enormous power that radiates from a person like a light, attracting others. An aura of selflessness makes saintly people shine so brightly that the essential goodness in others, even if deeply hidden, responds.

Before we seek realization, we have to get rid of our selfish self that grabs at everything, seeks constant gratification, and is ever ready to scheme the fulfillment of its own desires. A mind that is ever engaged in scheming without the practice of surrender to the divine will is so out of balance that no single exercise will remedy it. Serving others selflessly – losing oneself and taking delight in helping others – is the best preparation for meditation.

Selflessness can be cultivated if it is our ideal, even though at first we may not be able to avoid the ego patting itself on the back for every little effort. If we are sincere, we will try again and again to loosen the grip of the desire for self-gratification. The next phase may be acting from a sense of duty. But if we keep the mind focused on our goal of selflessness, we will know the difference. We must also accept where we are and not allow the ego to come in by the back door, claiming, "I am selfless."

Every work is the same. In the Bhagavad Gita, Krishna says, "Whatever obligatory action is done, O Arjuna, merely because it ought to be done, abandoning attachment and also the fruit, that renunciation is regarded as pure" (18, verse 9). The value is in the dignity of the person, the honesty with which the job is performed and the extra service given. This is the essence of Karma Yoga, to act but to leave aside attachment and the desire for rewards.

When I was at Sivananda Ashram, there was a famous medical surgeon on holiday. He said, "Swamiji, I'm going to retire early so I can spend the rest of my life here and I will be completely at your service."

Gurudev said, "How long are you here?"

"Another six weeks."

And Gurudev said, "Then why not start today?"

And he said, "Very well Swamiji. What should I do?"

"You can start by cleaning the latrines."

That was the last we saw of him. This particular work was not for him and he had no use for a guru who asked him to renounce his status.

When we have accepted an obligation, for example to do a specific kind of work, then we simply do it because it needs to be done. If we say, "I don't like this or I like that better," we are catering to our likes and dislikes. Ask yourself if the spirit of the work, the true giving, is there. Instead of waiting for somebody to say, "You were wonderful and I'm so grateful to you," your reward is knowing that you have done your best.

If we do service without self-gratification, we expand beyond ourselves. I think in our modern times we particularly need that. If I serve only myself I create a small world, and self-centeredness can be one of the most destructive forces. If I include you, then you are part of my world and my world becomes larger. Through service we learn to see the Divine in others. By being generous, we develop purity of mind.

Selflessness helps you to do the greatest good. Even if you are not self-realized, but if you somehow know there is an inner Light, try to kindle it in yourself and in other people too. That will strengthen and clarify your knowing. The highest knowledge is knowledge of this inner Light. Once you recognize it, then the greatest good you can do is to help others to find it. Do not support their weaknesses so they will like you better or be nicer or accept you. That is like an indirect stealing from the Divine.

It would be fine if we could change everyone else to make the world a better place. But this better world starts with each one of us. "Daily we must die," said St. Paul. Daily we must die to the urges that selfishness imposes on us. It is a hard and strenuous fight. Constant awareness sounds simple but carrying it out is a continuous struggle. In the practice of awareness, the mysteries of the mind are discovered, and so are the subtleties of the ego.

We start to understand that every thought and action, no matter how small, is part of the whole. The more we become capable of acting from a less selfish place, the more we come into harmony with the divine law. Divine law can be seen at work in all spiritual paths. While the symbols that express it may differ from culture to culture, the aim is the same – the oneness of our human consciousness with Cosmic Consciousness.

Let yourself be guided by how to put this knowledge into practice. The unselfish desire to serve, to help others, will pave the road. The divine force will then work through you. Repeated experience will bring about the awareness that God, the Light, Energy, works through you. Service of others then becomes worship. Selfless work becomes love manifest.

3 Facing the Ego

I'D LIKE TO TELL YOU a beautiful, ancient Chinese story that shows how renunciation works.

There was once a bell maker who wanted to make the most splendid sounding bell so that everybody would know that he had made the finest bell in the world. But every time he started, something terrible would happen – the metal would crack, a stone would roll into the mixture, and once a little animal even jumped into the pot. No matter how hard he tried, his bells were never perfect. He was so obsessed with the idea of being a great man who made the most fantastic bell that his wife deserted him and he eventually ran out of money.

Alone and poor, he was forced to give up and do something else just to make a living. One day when he was much older (and the power of his ego had worn down), he noticed some little village children playing outside his window. He felt inspired to gather together his old scraps of metal and make a row of tiny bells for each of them, tuning each set of bells slightly differently. The children were delighted. Soon people were coming from far and wide asking, "Who made these bells? These are the sweetest, most melodic sounds we've ever heard."

This story applies to all of us. The moment we want to be the famous bell maker – or saint or yogi – we will not succeed. When we want to do something for the love of God or to attain Cosmic Consciousness, it doesn't matter if anybody else knows.

What needs to be renounced is the control of the ego. Whenever we want to be famous or powerful, to be in a leading position or to control other people, whenever we are possessive or driven by compelling forces, that is the ego and its desires. As you do spiritual practice, you will come face-to-face with the ego, and it will fight back fiercely. You may have to resort to prayer to ask for the strength and courage needed to be honest with yourself. I noticed in my early life as a swami that I was developing the subtle thought, "I'm the *sanyasi* and you're the worldly people." So, I look off my orange robe and started to wear ordinary clothes. I didn't want to advertise myself. If you start to observe that you chant better when someone else is in the meditation room – stop, leave, come back and chant alone. The game we play with ourselves, sometimes unconsciously, is wanting to impress an audience, in this case with our great spirituality. It happens in every corner of daily life, too – "Look what a good cook I am!" "Look how many leaves I've raked compared to the others!"

Possessiveness is another area to investigate. Possessiveness means you are also possessed, whether by material things or by ideas – because the mental and material levels are not entirely separate. We cannot renounce something material unless we renounce it in the mind first. And we may have pockets of possessiveness that we're unaware of. If we are possessive of a person – husband, wife, children, friends – we prevent the other person from being what he or she ought to be – himself or herself. And this is not love. It is then much better to openly admit, "I have a need, which at the moment I am incapable of renouncing. To be honest, I need you." It is then up to the other person to decide whether or not to fulfill your needs, but at least you are not misleading them.

If you have deep feelings for a person, ask yourself how possessive you are. How many "becauses" do you attach to your love of that person? "I love you ... because you get a lot of work done ... because you help me ... because you give me emotional satisfaction." At least reverse the "because" to something positive: "I love you … because of your sincerity … because of what we have in common ..." rather than seeing what you can get out of them. This is especially important for anyone aspiring to be a spiritual teacher. Otherwise, you use people.

Love grows in the sunlight of renunciation best because it is unhampered, unhindered. In all paths of life, if we want to have harmonious relationships with others we have to renounce possessiveness and jealousy and preserve our energy for whatever it is we really want to do. So renunciation is necessary. If you really love, you will have to renounce self-gratification and emotional security. Sometimes it may even mean renouncing companionship because you understand that you may not have that much to give to another person. You may be attached only to an appearance of a relationship.

We also have to renounce our fantasies because

they are self-created, and if you have a powerful mind those fantasies can manifest later when you no longer want them. Instead of fantasizing, clarify. Face yourself and look at your needs. As long as you have needs, acknowledge them and find different ways to satisfy them that will not be harmful to yourself or dishonest to anyone else.

False modesty, false humility, false pride, self-pity – these are all dangerous games that need to be recognized and let go of. Trace them to their very roots, to the particular personality aspect that generates them. If you are compelled by jealousy, trace it back to the root of inferiority. Deal with that feeling, bring it to awareness. Do the same for any behaviour or emotion that seems beyond your control. The power is neutral. And the power that now keeps you bound can be redirected to something more beneficial, to your Higher Self. You can change stubbornness, which can be a real stumbling block on the spiritual path, into willpower, which can help support you in any creative endeavour.

Yoga is a path of liberation. You cannot force renunciation, but you can be determined to be liberated from anything that keeps you prisoner. When you kindle and nourish the desire to be free, you redirect the power from the greed of the compulsion and give energy to your personal path of liberation.

4 The Divine Path

THERE ARE TWO REALITIES – the reality of the world as it is and the reality of the awareness of your mind. It is quite a job to courageously face the facts of the world and yet aim for Higher Consciousness. We have to remember that the Divine protects us, but we have to stick to the Divine. When I made the decision to go to India, I knew in my inner being what I was looking for and that if I kept my intention straight I would not be disappointed. In the Christian teachings Jesus said, "If you ask your Heavenly Father for bread, He will not give you stones."

Do you know what the spiritual path really is – how many curves, how many windings, how many ups and downs? How do you know you are still on the path or if you have trailed off a little, or even gotten lost entirely? Your spiritual development will constantly undergo changes. The modern word for this is progress. Make sure that it is progress. Often changes come in disguise and we don't recognize them for what they are. We act on appearances without really understanding what is behind the appearances.

There was a time when you were safe within your mother's womb. Then, at one point, you had to leave that very cozy place where everything was taken care of, only to find yourself in this big wide world, not understood at all. You separated yourself from your mother's womb to establish your own life because you are a being that has its own consciousness. On the spiritual path, it is the same. You may be living in the cozy surroundings of home and family, career or business – all in a neat package and seeming to be quite secure. Why should anybody leave this? But progress on the spiritual path demands a separation from what has been.

When you begin your spiritual journey, at first you want only to be inspired. You may collect pictures and images, or read articles and entertaining books because you have nothing yet to contribute yourself, so you are gathering in your nourishment. Then you learn to stand on your own two feet and try to walk, and you may find it very shaky. Some try a little bit too early, and some are so afraid that they never want to make the attempt. But eventually you have to become independent and develop your ability to think. You can't depend on a teacher to demand discipline from you. You grow spiritually only when you understand what you can gain from this kind of work. At one point you have to take off your baby shoes, knowing the Divine requires a more developed human being to help with the work at hand.

We go through psychological and emotional processes that make us capable of connecting with the Divine. I heard Swami Sivananda once say to someone who felt dejected and separated from the Divine, "Ha! What did you do?" And the man said, "I didn't know what to do." Sivananda sat up straight and said emphatically, "You should have shaken a fist to the sky and said, 'Lord, you ought to listen! Come and help!'" I remember my great surprise when Sivananda, this tall and portly man, shook his fist at the sky. To explain himself, he added, "It's better to be angry at God than to turn your back."

Don't turn your back on the Divine. Stay involved. I remembered this and sometimes, over the years, would complain bitterly, "Why do you do this to me? Why didn't you stand by and remind me?" But when I became aware, I also learned to say thank you to my Higher Self.

Think about what your next step will be. How will you go about it? In any successful strategy, you have to give it everything you've got. We often think that on the spiritual path things are a little unfair. But, business is worse. And for what results? A materially rich life may look glamorous, but if the stock market crashes or the housing market tumbles, what have you gained? Do you have anything that you can fall back on? So that kind of security is very undependable. Keep your eyes open and don't get too engrossed in greed. Greed is something that needs to be trimmed back very early, like fruit trees. Perhaps it sounds accusing to use that term greed, but find out where "I want" ends and where greed begins. What is the motivation behind your desire? Who do you want to impress? If you impress the Most High, what else would you need?

To move on to your next phase, you need to shift from the outer guru to the inner guru, or what Jesus called "the kingdom of God within." It means quieting the emotions and really listening. When you need the guidance most, it is available – but you have to look for it.

Once you see the tremendous opportunity that life gives you to cooperate with the law of spiritual evolution, you will want to increase your efforts in personal development. Divine law has a specific application for each individual, suited to the karmic situations of our unique paths, but the overall purpose of life is the same for everyone. If you accept the challenge of evolution of consciousness, you will find that you have much greater equanimity to face whatever life offers. The option is always open to either cooperate with evolution or to resist the divine plan. If you make the choice to cooperate, you will undoubtedly experience increased peace and happiness.

5 What Does Enlightenment Mean to You?

RATHER THAN READING about enlightenment, each person has to clarify what he or she understands it to be. I would say that the more you know yourself, to that degree you are enlightened. If you really know yourself, you might know that you are not able to put everything into perfect action to the satisfaction of other people. But you are not here to please other people, to project an image. Enlightenment in that sense has as many levels as awareness.

The other term we can use is liberation. If you can liberate yourself and if you welcome anybody who helps you to liberate yourself from your limitations, you have already achieved a degree of understanding. There is no enlightenment without understanding. But if you immediately shrink back and react instantly when someone points out a weakness, you can be sure your ego is involved. Give yourself time to overcome that spontaneous, immediate reaction. You have to accept your reactions, but you don't want to carry them around for the rest of your life. You also have to accept your own divinity.

In other words, you first have to honestly admit where you are. If you don't know yourself, how can you be enlightened? Naturally your understanding of yourself will become more than a psychological knowing. You will become more open to divine inspiration and eventually to a wisdom that radiates from other sources to which, by your own efforts, you have made yourself available.

Liberation is an ongoing process, not an end state. It is a refinement, which language cannot express fully. It is like going down into a mine and finding diamonds. In their original, rough state, the diamonds are not beautiful and sparkling, and you may not even recognize them at first. They have to be cleaned, cut and polished. On the individual human level, cutting and polishing is the process that may seem to grind away your strength, energy, mental and emotional powers and endurance. But, upon reflection, the same events that could wear you down can actually contribute to greater clarity if you have the goodwill to observe the potential and to learn about yourself. Besides goodwill, you need to take action based on what you learn, and to recognize that there is wisdom in insecurity. All the senses have to be sharpened and developed to grow to a point of being truly useful. And we need to develop the sense of discrimination.

The path of liberation is an extremely difficult one. Different incidents will occur and as we tackle one area, we lose sight of another. When we are unskilled, we may use an axe when we need a fine scalpel. Learning takes time, and before we've learned one thing the next is already demanding our attention. How do we retain what we have already learned? It's not so different from trying to keep track of essential information in our modern information age when there is a barrage of input. We may think we need to specialize, but the moment we do we lose the input that may be relevant at some later date.

In the beginning it may appear impossible to manage this challenge of continuous learning, but again we have to look at an example from ordinary life. When we learn to drive a car, there are so many aspects to pay attention to – the handling of the car itself, the mechanical side, looking into the rear-view mirror, watching the street and the traffic. In the beginning it feels as if we're trying to be in too many places at once. Yet eventually driving becomes easy and smooth. What seemed impossible is achieved. It is the same on the path of liberation. Awareness will expand.

Self-reflection is very important. You may do mantra, meditation, Hatha Yoga, all of the spiritual practices, but if it doesn't settle in the depths of the mind, the lotus will not make even one shoot. Many gymnasts and figure skaters move beautifully; why don't they have realization? Reflection is essential. Any practice will have little result if it becomes an automatic routine. Use mantra chanting to express your emotions and as a way to let go of your intellect. Say to the Divine, "Here I am. You have given me these feelings. I have not handled them right. I need help." That is where humility comes in. If you don't have humility, somebody else will have to come along and humiliate you in front of others. If that happens, instead of getting angry, see if you can thank that person for being Divine Mother's instrument in liberating you from your monkey mind.

The power that we obtain through mantra or meditation is neutral, and what you do with this power is entirely your decision and your responsibility – an awesome responsibility. You will come to the edge more than once in your spiritual life where you can switch this power into the opposite. And this is why your commitment to your spiritual path is so very important. In proportion to your commitment, grace will sustain you. If the ego takes over, your so-called enlightenment means nothing. All the power that is acquired – and many people have very strong, powerful personalities – is hooked into the ego and self-will. So the responsibility is entirely the individual's. Sticking to your commitment means really dealing with your ego and self-will. It's as simple as that. And there is nobody and no power that can release you from that responsibility.

2 KUNDALINI YOGA: THE FOUNDATION

6 The Powerhouse

WHEN I'M ASKED to define Kundalini Yoga in simple terms, I usually ask the questioner to start by investigating "energy." When do you use the word? What do you mean by it?

We can think about energy in ordinary terms. You have probably seen big dams with power stations, where rivers are regulated and their power used to produce electricity. This electricity travels through cables to various places – from tiny villages to towns to huge metropolitan areas. Yet, wherever you are, you cannot access the electricity until you request it for your individual house. If you decide to hook up, you probably know why you want the electricity – for light, for cooking and heat, and for running your electronic equipment. How does the energy move from outside to inside? A big converter outside the house directs the electricity into the house and into every room. You can even decide where you want your power outlets.

Now let's take the same illustration to a cosmic level. In this case, you cannot see the power station; you may just have a feeling that there must be something else – a source. If you look at yourself, you know that you have a nervous system with electro-chemical charges – positive and negative. So power must be located in your body somewhere. Think about the spine and how the nerves extend out from this centre to different areas of your body. If you look at an anatomy book, you can see that the brain makes billions of connections, and these connections result in your ability to think and perceive and function. Just as the power station on a big river in the country eventually leads to a small place like your house, it is the same within you – there is a beginning place and there is a destination. And if you follow this path, you will see that all along the way you are involved in a marvelous and complex process.

You may begin to ask questions. What is the difference between mind and brain? When my brain dies, what happens to the energy? Physicists tell us that energy cannot be destroyed. Energy manifests through many different shapes and forms, and provides power for action. But for what purpose? As a human being, I am powered by something. How did the power get there?

There are various theories about our origin, and while they cannot be scientifically proven at this time, there are indications. If the universe started from a Big Bang, as astronomers hypothesize, it would be difficult to accept that human beings suddenly existed with fully developed brains. Certain religious groups are convinced that this is true and believe that human beings are a special creation of God. Then we would have to ask, "What is God?" If human beings are the special creation of the greatest power we can conceive of, it would be a sad state of affairs that we aren't more perfect.

It is a more adventurous hypothesis to think that evolution takes place, and that we move toward a perfection that already exists within ourselves, but which – like truth – we have to discover. And we do that in stages. For some people, it is easier to accept the hypothesis that there is a cosmic intelligence rather than a single God directing this course of evolution, because everything that is created has a certain intelligence. Just think of the fruit fly with an entire digestive system, a whole perceptual system and a pair of wings, all within its tiny body. In the life span of a single human being we cannot witness the whole course of evolution, but if we take a long-range view we can see how evolution must have taken place – right back to the point of a single cell splitting.

And today we find nuclear physicists in the same neighbourhood as people who can't read and write. How is this possible? Perhaps it is a mistake to believe that all people evolve together. But even if they did – and we shall never rule out any possibilities – how would it be possible to observe that process in the short span of a human life?

We evolve spiritually through our own personal efforts to understand the power that keeps us alive, the power that makes our minds work. As we grow in awareness, we start to understand more of that cosmic power. In India the name given to that power is Kundalini. In Greece it is called the "soul." Nobody has seen either. We can't always see everything, but just as in physics, we can see the traces. By starting to get to know ourselves and tracing the events of our lives, we will begin to see ourselves on a different scale than we are used to. Hereditary and environmental influences are not denied, but does that mean we have to limit ourselves to those influences or think that we are just the product of something?

Ask yourself many questions, and always be willing to challenge your own answers. How does a mind – which itself cannot be found and seen – function? What makes the mind work? Where does the mind get its power? These could be the first questions to pursue. And as you become stronger at looking at possibilities, you may accept the challenge of discovering the mystery deep within yourself of that innate power that some people call Kundalini.

Electricity is a neutral power: it can be put into service or it can electrocute. It has to be understood that the cosmic power is also neutral. We are responsible for how we allow our power to manifest. We cannot just run wild. You don't know how much power you have in your mental world until you allow this power to manifest properly. You may eventually discover that there are many different powers connected to mind. Intelligence is just one power and it manifests in varying degrees – from a faint glimmer to the enormous power of the genius, yet it is still the same energy.

The powers of the mind are awesome. We can use these neutral powers to understand the mind's own workings and how its powers are acquired. Energy, by whatever name we call it, is neutral. It is the responsibility of the individual how the power is used. Who judges if the energy is used rightly or wrongly?

Your own conscience. When our innate love is overruled, problems begin.

The study and practice of Kundalini Yoga can help us develop all of our potential and make us free and independent. At first, though, we need help because we don't have enough discrimination and awareness to use this power wisely. We are like sleepwalkers who need to wake up. In ordinary life we often do not notice the succession of happenings that lead to a result, but yogis, by their sense of observation, see that nothing happens without due preparation. Part of the training in Kundalini Yoga is to train the mind and the emotions to accept the facts as they are, without the emotional colouring that wants to see them differently.

Most people carry around the heavy burdens of emotional pain – resentment, dashed hopes, revenge, bitterness – emotions that have not yet been purified. These emotions are a dangerous starting point. With Kundalini Yoga we have to lay a foundation in our lives; otherwise we become confused. The mental and emotional garbage has to come to the surface and be dealt with. This is the process of character building, which is essential for any spiritual path, no matter what name you give it. The first cakra is pure energy: What are you going to do with it? You have to learn to use your own thinking power to the best advantage.

People often reject discipline without realizing that success in any field demands hours of practice. Without discipline in spiritual pursuits, the central nervous system doesn't have a chance to adjust and grow with the increased demand. It would be like putting a high voltage into a small bulb – it is bound to explode. In unusual Kundalini manifestations, there is often a strong element of self-will. Without a foundation in character building, the power can become a curse instead of a blessing. If you are learning to fly an airplane you have to learn how to take off and, just as importantly, how to land safely. It is the same with the path of Kundalini. Training is needed to learn to focus attention, sharpen discrimination and practise recall.

In the original Kundalini texts, the powers of the *cakras* are described in ways that may sound exaggerated and fantastic to people living in our time – for example, the power to render oneself invisible, the power to enter another's body, the power to create and destroy worlds. But these powers do indeed exist.

To become invisible, the first step is to see your own insignificance. You have to overcome the desire to be the centre of attention. This means overcoming self-importance and the desire to project a particular image out to others. When you are not caught up in the need to be seen and heard, that energy can come back to you to be used differently.

Entering another's body means entering the body of knowledge of another, the world that the person has created for himself or herself. When we are not self-centred, we can listen without interpreting their words through our experience. To do this, we need self-control in speech and the ability to keep silent.

Creating and destroying worlds: Think of the worlds you create by sweet talk or harsh talk, critical talk or coarse talk. By the same power you can destroy those worlds and create new ones. The power of speech to create and destroy worlds is of great importance. When you refine your expression, you can cultivate the right kind of desires and begin to express divine thoughts that will benefit others.

The Kundalini system is a very straightforward and direct path that expresses eternal truth; it is alive now. *Cakra* means "wheel" and wheel implies movement. So you want to move from the position where you are now in your personal development to something more elevated and intense. You can do this by reflecting on how you have learned in the past and what you could do differently. Where do you want to go? What do you want to achieve?

One of the greatest powers we have, although it is often not recognized, is the power of choice. With our mental power, we can choose to be kind, understanding and helpful, or jealous, envious and destructive. We can choose to give or to steal. The polarity is within us, and we first have to recognize it and then take responsibility for both the positive and negative ways we handle our power.

So ask yourself: What power am I engaging? What power am I loosening? If you have no control over it, what good is it? You have to go through life with awareness, thinking things through. Self-discipline and foresight are needed. If you want the power of Kundalini, you have to think it through. How do you use the powers you already have? Only you are responsible for your actions.

7 Symbolism of the Elements

WE LIVE IN A WORLD of fundamental elements – earth, water, fire, air, space. In the Kundalini system, each *cakra* has a corresponding element. You can gain an expanded awareness of your inner world by reflecting on the elements in the external world and asking how they exist within your own body and mind. Start by writing down your associations with earth, water, fire air, space, and then reflect on how these words relate to you personally. The following framework may be useful as a guide to exploring the symbolism of the elements through the *cakras*.

In the first *cakra*, the Muladhara, the element represented is earth. Just as earth supports life and growth, our personal growth is an ongoing process. This refers not just to physical growth but also to the growth of understanding and intelligence and the use of the senses. Through life experiences we grow a body of knowledge, which is an ongoing process.

The second *cakra*, the Svadisthana, is related to water and the imagination. What do we do with this fluidity of possibility? In the Divine Light Invocation, we can imagine people moving up into the source of all

Light, an ocean of Divine Light. This ocean symbolizes unlimited bliss: *ananda*. But to reach it we have to control the waves of the mind.

Our imagination is like water and can range from murky to very clear. Like water, the imagination can be very supple and smooth, stagnant or flowing, gushing or falling in torrents, and it will have the respective effect in our lives. Visions of Light arise only when we are properly focused and when the mantra is rooted. Mantra will purify the waters of the imagination.

Fire is the element of the third *cakra*, the Manipura, related to the sense of sight and to the emotions. Just as fire radiates heat, the fire of knowledge radiates wisdom. The classical saying in yoga is that "ignorance is burned in the fire of wisdom." Fire also has a tremendous power of destruction and the fires of passion can burn on many levels. When we are angry, we "see red." We can experience the animal heat of sexual passion and the constant burning for more. Burning desires can be a great flame or they can be embers smoldering in the unconscious.

The third *cakra* controls sight. Ask yourself what sight means. What is insight? Can you see in the mind's eye? When you have spiritual insight, all of the pairs of opposites – pain and pleasure, hate and love – are understood as fluctuating emotions. The eyes can flame with jealousy or burn with criticism or anger. If you want your eyes to emanate clear Light, offer the pairs of opposites back to the Divine in return for Divine Love.

The element of the fourth *cakra*, the Anahata, is air. This *cakra* is also related to touch. We breathe without having to convince ourselves that we breathe, even though air is invisible. We need air to produce sound – without air we cannot speak, chant or even whisper. The purest breath is that which produces the mantra. Air, with its qualities of fleetness, lightness and invisibility, cannot be grasped and held onto.

In the fifth *cakra*, related to the sense of hearing, *akasha* (sometimes translated as "space" or "ether") is the element. *Akasha* is the power of flight and transparency. Is it possible to become so transparent that you would not cast a shadow? What could be meant by the ethereal body and the ethereal region? How can you make your mind as wide as the sky? When we concentrate, meditate, contemplate, we open to a vastness beyond suggestion, an openness to the past, present and future.

Harmony comes when the elements are beautifully blended together. All five elements create an interplay of forces, and when transmuted, they have transcendental aspects that lead to an extraordinary power. Understanding the symbolism of the elements can lead to a realization of how everything is always there for us at any time, in any place.

8 A Taste for the Divine

IN THE KUNDALINI SYSTEM, imagination is governed by the second *cakra*. This *cakra*, or level of consciousness, also controls the sense of taste and desire. The relationship between imagination, taste and desire is worth investigating.

Imagination swims in the waters of our thoughts and ideas and is open to stimulation from wherever it comes. Imagination gives birth to desire, and desires – especially those for pleasure – seek gratification.

In visual representations of the second *cakra*, the imagination is pictured as a *makara*, a mythical alligator-fish with a mouth big enough to swallow almost anything. Its teeth symbolize greed or a desire to hold on.

But even the imagination cannot hold on to everything at once. Our thinking process can be so fast that many thoughts are not even caught. Some ideas will arise that stimulate the imagination, while others will pass by. We also cannot manifest every potential idea. As human beings, we are limited in our expression.

If an idea does capture the imagination, we have to activate our innate intelligence to discriminate whether it is better to let the idea go or to hold onto it and pursue it to greater understanding. It is almost like learning to develop a taste for healthy food. What will benefit us in the long run? Different situations will call for different choices. But recognize that the power of choice is ours. We have to take charge of the direction of the imagination through awareness. And because we do not have complete awareness, we can also rely on intuitive perception – those glimmers of understanding that are not necessarily clear, but that can be interpreted and worked with to bring about clearer understanding.

Left unattended, imagination can be misleading. A vivid imagination can lead to building up unrealistic hopes and expectations. When the imagination goes unchecked and uncontrolled, it can also create unnecessary fears. Imagination is the source of much self-inflicted pain. For example, in a relationship, people often envision their life as a romantic film. Imagination interferes with the reality. There are two real people, and you have to come around to accept yourself as you are in order to be able to accept the partner that you want to be involved with. You also have to accept your partner the way he or she is.

There are numerous exercises to cultivate the imagination, including the practice of worship. Through spiritual practice and study, you feed the imagination spiritual food. The *makara* will eat anything and, with time, can develop a taste for the Divine.

If you give as much time as possible every day to the Divine, you will increase your taste and desire for the Divine. And your desire for the Divine, even if it is fulfilled to a very small degree, will nourish you for a long, long time. Once you have a taste of the Divine, you will know there is nothing better, nothing more desirable. You taste heaven itself. The point of meditation and study is eventually to give you that taste of Divine nectar and ambrosia, which is much more satisfying than the sugar candy of all your other desires.

The Divine wants to give us what is real and lasting, but instead of accepting this gift, we throw tantrums and hold onto our artificially coloured candies. We cannot be given more until we let go. Our hands need to be empty to receive, then we can overflow and give to others. You can give the physical body what it needs, but detach yourself from it. Don't become overly involved. When you give the body food, don't make a big deal out of it. Don't worship food or make diet another god. Whatever your understanding of human love is, don't make that another god, either.

Beyond gratification of desires is the greater adventure of expanded awareness, which leads to experiences that the imagination cannot even dream up.

People sometimes ask me whether a spiritual seeker should have an exclusive taste for the Divine or rather a taste for doing good toward others in the world. It is never an either/or question. To integrate the spiritual, we have to bring quality into our life as we live it. We each have to define what we mean by "quality" and decide what kind of person we want to be, because one world feeds on the other. If you don't live according to your ideals or values in your daily life, that inattention will show up in your spiritual life. If you are very dedicated in your spiritual life, that dedication will filter into your daily life. It's not either the world or the Divine, but the interaction.

It's up to each of us to develop a balanced, healthy diet for the imagination, a taste for quality and compassion, that can then manifest and help create the kind of world we want to live in.

9 Seeking Awareness Through Hatha Yoga

FOR MOST PEOPLE, it is impossible to comprehend the tremendous phenomenon of the whole cosmos in which we find ourselves. Yet somehow we have to form a relationship to the cosmos or find our place in it. You can begin to gain more understanding of your relationship with the world around you by practising Hatha Yoga.

Hatha Yoga is a good beginning for many people because it involves the physical world that we know exists and that we can understand. Like any practice, it is effective if you apply what you learn and stay with it. You also have to find out what you want to gain from Hatha Yoga, as it is a complex system for the development of the whole human being. You need a certain goal beyond physical strength, beauty and agility.

Hatha Yoga is tremendously precise. Each asana can lead to insights, and all of the asanas are interconnected. The whole system is part of the larger Kundalini system, a path to Higher Consciousness.

Trikonasana, the asana where triangles are

formed with your own human body, is an excellent pose for discovering more about relationship and interconnection. A triangle, a simple geometrical form, is also a powerful symbol.

Scientists today say that the universe can be understood mathematically. Thousands of years ago in India, the same idea was expressed slightly differently through a *yantra* (or mandala) called Sri Yantra. The Sri Yantra is composed of many triangles – a triangle within a triangle, another triangle within a triangle, within a triangle. It's like a maze. In the tiniest triangle at the centre, there is just a dot. The collection of triangles is sometimes called Divine Mother's castle, symbolizing the Cosmic Energy giving birth to creation. The dot in the very centre means that all power emanates from there.

The ascending triangle, where the tip points up, is symbolically the individual's approach to this Greater Power. But there would be no reason for reaching up if there was not something also coming down. So the descending triangle symbolizes grace or the concern of the Divine for what it has created. The devotee who is seeking Higher Consciousness can use the *yantra* as a map. The same idea is expressed in the two triangles of the Heart Lotus in the Kundalini system, where an ascending and a descending triangle intersect to form a star. When you make the effort to reach toward the divine power, it moves down to meet you halfway. You may think you have to do it all yourself, but that is not so.

In the Triangle pose, it is important to have your base aligned and to know what you are aiming for. Then you can also observe what comes back as a response.

The Triangle posture emphasizes the three parts of the interplay of forces: dependency, interdependency and interaction. As an individual, you need to realize that you are not living in the world entirely on your own. Nobody does. Wherever you stand, you have to admit that you didn't make the ground you stand on. So you are constantly depending on something else. Study your dependencies carefully and find out also where you have the wrong kind of dependency.

What about interdependency? Can you recognize interdependency in your relationships with your loved ones or with your colleagues? Interdependency means receiving the response back. With interaction, think about how various elements interact to create a precise situation. When you start a fire, for example, it depends on three things – the fuel, the oxygen that feeds the flame, and the process of your lighting the fire. Another example would be the air, the flute and the flute player – you need all three to produce the melody. In the same way, there is an interaction between you, the teachings and the teacher, and the result is very important.

We often want to be independent, but it is impossible. We depend on a healthy body, we depend on a healthy mind, and we depend on the interaction of the two.

In geometry, the triangle is the most stable shape and has the most tremendous strength of any form. Once you connect with that strength – and keep in mind that just as in the Sri Yantra, you can put your triangle into a triangle into a triangle – you give yourself the message that there is nothing to fear. Gradually you can make your way back to the very centre of your own being, discovering the inner source from which the power emanates. The innate power that was unknown to you can now be realized and used effectively. Instead of being a sleepwalker, you become a very aware person.

It is this awareness that you should seek through the practice of yoga. As yogis and yoginis, the focus should not be on perfectionism or striving for recognition – those are cultural or social ideas. The focus should be on the Divine, on using your body as a spiritual tool. Think about what a marvelous tool the body is, and how unfortunately in our ignorance we may have abused it in the past. Through the practice of Hatha Yoga, you can conquer fears and broaden your self-knowledge. Balancing physically in a pose can be the start of seeing that with effort, practice, attention and goodwill, you can achieve balance in other areas of your life.

10 The Path

WHEN WE THINK of the environment, we usually think of the planet we live on and the ground it provides us. In the Kundalini system, each *cakra* is associated with one of the elements, and "earth" is the element of the first *cakra*, the Muladhara, which controls the creative power and is the seat of the latent Kundalini.

Think about the creative power of earth. What is growing? What is grounded? What is rooted? What strength do you draw from? Look at the manifestation of your own creation. See how your concepts create your own little world – your mental world, your emotional world, your spiritual world. What have you created for yourself?

The earth provides the ground for growing. Each of us is growing in an ongoing process, which we can call "the path." The path is nothing other than the process of our development toward greater awareness. The particular method that appeals to you – Christianity, Buddhism, etc. – is just a vehicle by which you travel this path.

What is your process of growth? The physical body obviously develops from childhood, but if you reflect on your life you will also see that you have grown in understanding, in intelligence, in accepting the world around you. You have grown in the use of your senses. Your body of knowledge to this point includes all that you have grown into, whether or not you have consciously entered a particular spiritual path.

We can expand the idea of the earth to include not only the physical earth that we walk upon, but also the ground of the body, the ground of the mind and the ground of the heart. You can observe what has grown in each area and ask what you want to grow.

On the yogic path, you can become grounded in the sacred word – the mantra or name of God. Your heart is the most precious soil. When the mantra is rooted in the heart, it will spread like a network of nerves throughout all the cells of your body, and the power will become grounded in your body. The mantra influences the consciousness of the cells, spiritualizing your body and also making the mind more flexible.

Having a flexible mind means remaining open to new and challenging ideas – expanding your awareness, increasing your intelligence and exercising all of your mental capacities. Just as plants are rooted in the earth, you have to discover which concepts have taken root in your mind. Many ideas are rooted in tradition, culture and family conditioning. Some of these concepts – fears, ambitions, desires – may be like rocks, preventing new growth from sprouting. Just as a gardener looks after the garden, you need to tend the garden of your mind – removing what obstructs growth, digging out the weeds and pruning back excess growth. As you dig into the ground of your own mind, you can examine which of your ideas are your own and which need rooting out.

YOUR INTELLIGENCE is not your ability to believe, but rather, your ability to test belief and manifest your knowledge in your own personal life. When you manifest your intelligence to a certain degree, you will break out of the shell of your self-created little world. At one point you will realize you are the creator of worlds, and that you can also destroy worlds – not the galaxy out there, or planetary systems, but the world that has been created by your mind. In other words, you can change what hasn't worked in your life or what has hindered the evolution of consciousness. You don't have to resent your past or criticize yourself, because you will start to understand that we all learn by trial and error.

Eventually when you fully explore the little world you have created around yourself, you can expand your horizons. People with true intelligence have enough clarity, insight and awareness to learn from the mistakes of others without making the same mistakes themselves. Even today, with all of our study of history, we have not yet learned to avoid war. We, as human beings, cannot seem to break out of this self-created limitation. The yogi must break out of his or her self-created limitations. That is the motivation in yoga.

Widen the horizon of your understanding. Know when to sow a seed, and watch to see it grow. It needs your concern, and love and attention. The seed will only sprout in the right conditions – good soil, light, water.

We can sow the seeds; the Divine makes them grow. You can pray for that growth. Have patience. The path is an ongoing process.

In the first *cakra*, the earth is symbolized by a square. This square is within a full white circle, which symbolizes completion. What would it mean to complete all the work you have come to do on Earth?

3 MIND & CONSCIOUSNESS

11 A Silent Revolution

LIFE THESE DAYS has become very complex. There is such an enormous input of information that our heads begin to whirl – we don't know what to do with it all. So first we need to take a good look at ourselves and ask, "How do I experience life?"

You can find out where you are by taking one step at a time in a process of clarification. What does mind mean to you? What does consciousness mean? And how would you combine and interweave these two ideas into living and making your living a true art? Can you put yourself on a course of evolution and cooperate with it, not leaving it to chance – wondering, will it work, will it not work? Can you take matters into your own hands and direct your life so that you can say, "Living is a particular art and I have made the best of it."?

The mind has many powers and when you train your mind, you will see that you can attain some remarkable achievements. What the mind creates, the mind can create again anytime. That which radiates from another source, however, which can be called "consciousness," cannot be attained at will. When we tap into that source, our life becomes so different, so enriched that we feel we have truly just begun to live.

Nourishing ourselves on the inside of our very being helps us to cope with the complexities and uncertainties of life, the helplessness we feel when we can't control world events. There are too many power structures. We cannot fight them all at once. They have been on Earth since humans started walking around trying to expand their territory, conquering other countries. It has always been the same. Perhaps the methods of war, politics and economics have changed, but the basic elements have always been there. People have wondered what they can do about their helplessness, and how they will survive, and where they will go from here. But often it is not until we are so hurt or feel such a sense of helplessness or emptiness that we begin to think deeply.

Does it have to be that way? Do we have to be clobbered by all these dramas that many of us have already experienced? Some generations lived through the time of the Depression. Others have been through world wars and know a different kind of life. But there is often little we can do outside ourselves to address these global issues, unless people group together to protest or start a revolution.

Sometimes, on an individual level, we can also have what I call "silent revolutions." The silent revolution is when you change on the inside, taking a new look at life and who you are. You may decide that life has to change, but you can't change the world. So what can you change? Only yourself, and you might be able to help change others – awakening them to the need for greater awareness. You can sharpen your intelligence. You can even cooperate with your own destiny. You don't have to wait until life breaks you down in pain. Pain is a great teacher and for some, it is the only teacher. But life doesn't have to be that way.

When you recognize and accept the gift of consciousness, you realize it's time to do something with it. That's when you get control over your life. You don't feel helpless, no matter what is going on in the world around you. And the inner security that so many people try to find through higher education, more money, greater social status, now comes through your own efforts.

The only question is, When are you going to start? Or for those of you who have started some time ago, but haven't done much, hoping everything would develop effortlessly by itself – I'm afraid it won't.

All truly great artists have done a lot of work and practice, not just keeping up their skills at a constant level but continually trying to increase them. Be an artist in your life. Increase the skills that you have. Discover new ones, and don't think for a minute that the limitations you have accepted to this point need to be accepted. Don't wait till destiny hits, and then you have to do something. Don't wait until the dramas come down and make you wake up. Look for the treasure in your own backyard. Expand your mind slowly into a region where you become aware of how great and vast your consciousness can really be.

12 Keys to Freedom

IF WE CAN SEE how much symbolism we use in daily life – consciously and unconsciously – it becomes clear how important it is to pay attention to symbolism in all areas. The clothes we wear, the colours we choose, how we sit, our gestures and mannerisms are all symbolic of who we are. They express something of our interior life. If you keep your eyes and ears open and are a good observer, you will see that much is revealed that is thought to be hidden. The conscious mind is so busy; it is always occupied, sidetracked, diverted, so it barely ever listens to the messages. If you want to know yourself, be open to everything possible.

Once you understand symbolism, the secrets of different cultures and religions also can start to open up. I studied the symbolism of Hinduism and Buddhism in India, Thailand and other cultures, and finally came full circle back to the Christian scriptures of my own culture. Suddenly everything fell into place. Reading, for example, the Book of Revelation literally, I could not make sense of it at all. But when I took time to study and understand the symbolic meaning, I found this text very closely linked to the Kundalini Yoga system.

In India, there are carvings and wall paintings on the temples and in the famous caves of Ajanta. The Divine images are not meant to be decorative, but rather to communicate knowledge in the most accessible way because written language had developed slowly and was available only to a few. And writing itself is symbolic. Each letter is an abstract symbol that combines with others to form a word. And behind each word is a myriad of ideas, open to interpretation by every reader. I think as long as we use words, the best we can do is to use symbol and metaphor.

Symbols have many levels and you have to stay with them until you begin to understand their meanings. When you increase your awareness through the study of symbols, you will recognize that your needs are more than just on the physical, emotional and intellectual levels. You will find out what enriches your life and what gives you a new incentive to live fully. The self-knowledge you gain will provide a wonderful protection against being manipulated by others and by yourself.

In the Eastern way of teaching, you are given as much opportunity to discover by yourself as possible. Only through that discovery comes the strength, the joy and the interest to pursue further. Listening, obedience and surrender are necessary in the beginning to develop receptivity. Once you are receptive, you become a self-generating force.

The emphasis in my teaching is on self-examination and self-inquiry. I use familiar Western terms, but in a kind of Eastern psychology that explores each person's individual symbolism and use of metaphor, and teaches the practice of awareness.

A walking meditation technique, which I now call Straight Walk, is tremendously symbolic from the very first step, and originated from an experience I had in Thailand. I was there visiting a monastery and the disciplinary Buddhist monk said to me, "Walk from here to there, observe everything, and tell me what you observe."

I put my foot out to take the first step and he said, "No, no, no. Back you go."

What did I observe? I started to go through the mechanics, lifting my foot up, putting it forward and walking.

Again he said, "No, go back," offering no help. In the West, we want to be spoon-fed. We want everything explained so we can understand it right away, and even then we cannot see it most of the time. In the East, you find out for yourself.

As I stood, I realized that when I was still, the weight of my body was evenly distributed and I was in a state of equilibrium. This state is symbolic of the equilibrium I sometimes felt in my life, but I knew that no one can stay in that position forever. Life is motion and development. So before I started, I realized that in order to move, I must make the decision to upset the equilibrium and change my situation.

When I expressed this insight, the monk let me take the first step. I observed how my weight shifted and my balance was thrown off. Once I completed the first step, I immediately began to take the second, but the monk stopped me. "No, no, you go back and start all over again."

Gradually I realized that when I brought my foot down and was ready to shift my weight, there was a split second when equilibrium was re-established. I understood that this was symbolic in life for re-establishing balance between any two steps, between two events or even between two thoughts. We have to recognize that the moment of balance exists in order to take the opportunity for rest and renewal. That is very important to understand and is usually missed in the West, because life is fast. We don't take the time to observe, and then we pay a high price.

Understanding and working with symbolism is a learning process where we find out for ourselves. Each of us can change our situation in life and live with more awareness. Symbolism is a key, but it is up to each person to put the key in the lock and open the door. That door leads to a new freedom. If you want it, it is all yours.

13 The Body Garden

DID YOU EVER LOOK at your body as if it were a garden? If you would take a walk through this unusual garden, you would discover something most beautiful and interesting. A good gardener watches the plants' growth quite regularly and with good intention, yet never interferes, instead trying to support when and where necessary. Relaxing in this way is most enjoyable and refreshing because you are walking through your body garden, getting a close look, putting attention where needed. And the body pays this kindness back manifold – in good health, strength and proper functioning.

Most people live in a hectic way, always rushing and racing. Yet what is accomplished does not match the price because this rushing is too demanding. The way of modern life has made us forget what life is really about. Have you ever asked what the purpose of your life is? Why you are here? What is the mysterious thing that we call mind? How does it function? And how does it function in relation to the body?

We may not realize how the restlessness of our thoughts and our emotions put the body under stress.

When we are angry, we breathe in a shallow way. When we laugh, our breath is staccato. When we are in peace and harmony, beyond the opposites of pain and pleasure, our breath is even. The constant desire for pleasure in numerous ways needs to be brought under control. The energy and the life-force can only be abused to a certain point, then the law of nature and the law of life close the door.

Body and mind are closely knit together. It may take time before the body reacts but when it does so in a disturbing way, it means there has already been a large amount of negative influences coming from the mind. False ideas, false images. They are like woodworms digging tiny little channels into the body. And when these are numerous and get away unchecked, the undermining activity brings a collapse in the physical – first, in those parts that are weak. The breakdown comes gradually but because we are unaware of the beginning, we may think it is sudden.

In the course of time, the influences of heat and cold, wind and rain make the hardest rock brittle. In the same way, the strongest health can break down if you don't care for your body. Mental and emotional stresses work on the human body, breaking down resistance over the course of time. What might be just temporary tiredness from lack of sleep or late hours may also be interpreted by the mind as weak health and susceptibility, and this thought can be absorbed until it actually manifests. The undermining takes place slowly unless we do something about it.

We need periods of rest and quiet – time for

ourselves to relax. In Savasana (the Corpse pose), we lie on the ground with all senses shut off. We can feel tension in our bodies, and we will also feel when we relax. First we die to the noise outside and then we hear the noise within our bodies, such as the blood singing in our ears or our heartbeat. To let the mind concentrate on the various parts of the body helps us to direct our thinking into these parts. But we need to relax the mind as well as the body. Can you relax your mind and still maintain awareness?

To learn to be quiet, to keep the body under control, helps us gradually to tune in with others. When we practise awareness in our daily lives and in our interactions with those around us, we can unlock the great creative forces within us.

When we are able to tune in by keeping our minds and our emotions quiet and under control, we become aware. We develop intuition. Within each of us there is an inner fountain that will overflow in the proportion to which we share. The greatest joy that we experience is the joy we share in the lives of others. Peace and harmony come to us when we bring peace and harmony to others. Who has not experienced an almost miraculous supply of energy when we are concerned for and helping someone else? And someday our practice will be rewarded with the experience of tuning in to that great force that gives life so abundantly.

In yoga, we wish to join our own consciousness with Cosmic Consciousness. There is no prescription for how to think about this energy, and it will reveal itself in the degree to which you approach and open up toward a new understanding. Remember, "I am not the body. I am not the mind. I am eternal energy, ever renewing, ever pure."

14 Dreams: The Forgotten Language

DREAMS are sometimes thought of as the forgotten language of the unconscious. How can we remember the meaning of this language? In our waking state, we use words that we are most familiar with or words that best express ourselves. In our unconscious, this is even more the case. To learn the language, we have to study it.

The Eastern teachings consider the mind the sixth sense because the mind has one main function – to interpret events, emotions and perceptions. How does the mind interpret? It collects experiences in the memory, storing them for use at other times as points of reference. What is going on in your mind while you sleep? What is the interior life of your dreams?

In recalling dreams, we are seeing with the mind's eye, and that power can become very strong. Recalling dreams requires an effortless intensity – tension doesn't help. Being relaxed and sincerely wanting to know can help you recall the dream. If the dream was very involved, you may remember just the end of it. A simple way to start to investigate the dreaming mind is to write down your dream as soon as you wake up, and sign it, which implies that you've recorded it as accurately as you can. Start by writing whatever you can recall and more may come. Even if you remember only fragments, write them down. They can contain incredible insights.

Then write what you were most busy with the previous day – your conscious concerns. In a second paragraph, write a very quick initial interpretation of the dream. After this, select the main symbols, or "key words," from the dream and begin to write your associations. If a word has many different meanings to you, put them all down. Then, holding all this material lightly in your mind, try to find what the dream could mean.

As you work with your dreams, more meaning will emerge and you will become clearer about the one-third of your life spent sleeping, which is normally not within your awareness.

You can take it a step further, too. At the end of each week, write down each dream from memory without looking at them. This is a technique to train yourself to recall – a valuable tool for developing awareness, not just in the realm of dreams but in daily life. We want to be able to recall incidents as correctly as possible. As you become more courageous, you will be able to recall dreams that show you an undesirable picture of yourself. And if you can accept this picture, you can work with what the dreams are pointing out and make substantial changes to yourself. Suddenly, you may be able to recall events from your very early life.

Nothing is more fascinating than exploring what

is within ourselves. Observe the balance of your senses in dreams. Do you dream only in visual images? In black and white or colour? Can you hear somebody speak to you in a dream? Can you smell, taste or touch something? If you can bring all of your five senses in, you will sharpen your sense perceptions in daily life, which is how we perceive the world.

Working with dreams can lead us to the wisdom within – whether we call it the inner being, the guru within, the kingdom of God, the Absolute, nirvana, eternity. I call it "my Divine Committee," and it has done a terrific job of giving me direction and leading me to where I needed to go.

In the beginning, we are spiritual babies, and like babies, our walk is not very steady. We toddle around, we fall, we have to get up and try again. But eventually, we need to grow up and mature, so that those divine forces can work through us. We often say that we are only a channel for something higher, but let's be a channel that is well scrubbed! That is what the spiritual work does. If we open an unused water tap, little bits of rust and dirt and silt will come pouring out. Dreams are a marvelous way of telling us what kind of dirt is in the channel, how to recognize and remove it. As you collect and study your dreams, you will learn to trust this additional guidance from within yourself.

The language of dreams arises from our individual unconscious. Other people can only interpret our dream as if it were theirs. Learning our own forgotten language, we start to become actively involved in our unconscious life.

Finding out how the mind functions is easier through dreams than through all our conscious efforts, where the mind is the instrument that investigates itself. But in dreams we are not consciously manipulating the mind and the messages can come through more clearly. When we dream, the part that competes with intuition is silenced; therefore, dreams can guide us in furthering our own course of evolution.

If you look at your dreams in a year, you may be surprised at what you have already known. Dreams can keep us going and keep us nourished. Our inherent self-interest can be used in a most beneficial way – to get to know ourselves.

15 The Yoga of Light

I am created by Divine Light.
I am sustained by Divine Light.
I am protected by Divine Light.
I am surrounded by Divine Light.
I am ever growing into Divine Light.

MANY SPIRITUAL PRACTICES over the centuries have become separated from the original teachings. Mantra is one of them and the Yoga of Light is another. Light is used as a symbol in all religions, in all ancient texts. Jesus says in the New Testament, "I am the way and the Light." Wisdom is often called Light. It is very important to clarify what you mean personally when you use the term "Light."

Yoga is the Path of Light. In the practice of the Divine Light Invocation* we use the power of imagination to allow the Light to come in. Very rarely can the mind actually create an image that brings the power of Light, but it can open the door to the experience.

There are many exercises to help prepare you

for the Divine Light Invocation because it requires concentration, which is not everyone's greatest strength. It means concentrating on the various muscles of the body to produce maximum tension, concentrating on the breath, and practising the mantra of the Light sufficiently so that it resides in your heart. It takes a while before all the aspects of the Invocation will be properly comprehended and can be done in a flowing way. You need to concentrate on the physical movement, briefly focus on the individual or group of people being put in the Light, let the feelings from the heart flow in, and remain focused on the Light. All of this needs to come together like a dance, like a little speck of dust that dances in a ray of sunlight.

One of the preparatory exercises is to tense the various parts of the body in a smooth way so that the mind can shift to the breath. When that is done, the mantra has to be put into the heart by clarifying what it means to you.

You can prepare the imagination by visualizing a pond of lotuses and see one bud, tightly closed. Watch as the lotus slowly opens in the sun, and understand that it takes time to let the Light emanate from the Lotus of the Heart.

Visualize a pearl or a diamond and see light playing on it and eventually emanating from it. Bring all of the powers of your mind together to focus on that very small jewel, as if you could dissolve it entirely into Light.

Another preparation is to understand the words of the Divine Light Invocation mantra so fully that they become filled with the very substance of Light.

In between the practices it is important to keep the thought of Light active by seeing how Light plays a large part in daily life and communication. As you practise the Light Invocation, first as an exercise and then as a spiritual practice, it may entice you to think more about the Light in your life. You may start to see that Light is not just present in your waking state, but also in your dreams. Observing your dreams is of utmost importance.

Eventually you will experience your own body completely filled with Divine Light. It is one of the very important results of practising the Divine Light Invocation.

Then you realize that the physical body is more of an illusion than the body composed of Light. The expectation that one day you will experience the body as a mass of Light should be kept in the back of your mind. Think of your physical body as a product of imagination, and note any insights that help you feel your body being filled with Light.

If you are prepared to give of yourself in the Divine Light Invocation, and do so truly from the Light of your heart, you are yielding to a power that is beyond anything you can imagine.

To become aware of the Light in yourself it is absolutely necessary to maintain inner calm. You have to learn to cultivate understanding about how the Light works, which means overcoming the tendencies to be superficial, hasty or wrongly motivated. One of the most impenetrable screens to the Light is intellectual arrogance. Struggles with intense desires and struggles in accepting other people make the Light fade.

Tensing the muscles with proper coordination of the breath will help concentration. If attention is extended to the *prana*, symbolized in the subtlety of the breath, you will achieve increased effectiveness.

Gurus and images of the Divine can be put into the Light so their physical appearance fades into Light, a sign that the aspirant has gone beyond the need of images.

Holding the Light and exclusive focus on the Light is necessary for any kind of experience of the Light. At the start it is helpful to focus on any resentment until it is dissolved in the Light. The same can be done with intense desires. If there are more than one, they should be focused on individually until each one has dissolved in the Light before proceeding with the completion of the Light Invocation. Other strong emotions should be treated in the same way.

You must guard the Light in your heart – no matter how small – very carefully, very vigorously. You can never be too careful or too attentive.

INSTRUCTIONS FOR PRACTISING THE DIVINE LIGHT INVOCATION

Stand erect, feet shoulder-width apart.

Keep the eyes closed and focus them on the space between the eyebrows.

Lift the arms above the head at the same time as you smoothly and gradually tense the whole body, while you inhale. The arms should be kept straight and the tension maintained throughout the body.

Hold the tension and the breath. Mentally, repeat the Divine Light Invocation mantra.

I am created by Divine Light.
I am sustained by Divine Light.
I am protected by Divine Light.
I am surrounded by Divine Light.
I am ever growing into Divine Light.

Then slowly lower the arms as you exhale and relax.

Keep the eyes closed and use your imagination to see yourself standing in a shower of brilliant white Light. See the Light pouring down upon you, flowing into the body through the top of the head, filling your entire being.

Now, without raising the arms, keeping them at your side, tense the body and inhale.

Hold the tension and the breath.

Again, mentally repeat the Divine Light Invocation mantra.

I am created by Divine Light.
I am sustained by Divine Light.
I am protected by Divine Light.
I am surrounded by Divine Light.
I am ever growing into Divine Light.

Slowly exhale and relax.
With the arms beside the body, concentrate on feeling a warm glow of Light suffuse your entire body, outside as well as inside.
Acknowledge silently to yourself:

Every cell of this, my physical body, is filled with Divine Light.
Every level of consciousness is illumined with Divine Light.
Divine Light penetrates every single cell of my being, every level of consciousness.
I have become a channel of pure Light.
I am one with the Light.

The Divine Light Invocation is an exercise of will as well as an act of surrender.
Be receptive to the Light and accept that you are now a channel of Divine Light.
Express your gratitude with deep feeling.
Have the desire to share this gift with someone whom you wish to help.
Turn your palms forward.

You can now share the Divine Light with any friend or relative. Keep the eyes closed and visualize him or her standing before you.

Mentally open the doors of your heart centre and let the Light stream forth toward the feet of this person. See the Light encircling the person and spiraling upward in a clockwise direction, enveloping the body completely.

See the spiral moving high up into the sky, taking his or her image along with it.

Finally the person merges into the source of the Light and becomes one with the Light. You may even lift your head to follow the spiral of Light, keeping the eyes closed. When the person has passed from your view, relax and silently give thanks for having the opportunity to help someone in need.

4 KNOWLEDGE

16 Knowing Vs Believing

WE HAVE TO CLARIFY to ourselves what we believe versus what we really know. When we say, "I believe," we indicate that we don't know by personal experience. "I believe that I will go to heaven if I don't smoke, if I don't eat meat, if I don't drink, if I'm loyal to my spouse, if I don't lie." What I'm really saying is, "I don't know but I hope so."

Beliefs are usually based on the words of a person, or a scripture or school of thought that we consider an authority. We apply these words to ourselves because they appeal to us, and then we begin to believe they are true. We have no means of assuring ourselves of this truth, because, for example, the moment I go to heaven, I don't come back and tell you. Even if I found myself in heaven, how would I know whether it is a heaven I have dreamed up in my imagination? What do I know of heaven?

Every guru I met asked me to try, to test and to do. I was asked to suspend judgement only temporarily until I had my own experience, but I was never asked to simply believe. If you meet somebody who wants you to blindly accept his or her words as truth, I would be very careful.

You have a right to doubt, but doubt with discrimination, doubt with intelligence. Doubt must not become a back door for laziness – an excuse for not working on yourself. If you don't doubt, you may think you already know everything, erecting a wall of limitation that you then cannot go beyond. Always doubt that you have reached the ultimate goal, or the maximum development of your perceptions. We have to push out further and further beyond the current limits of our mental and perceptual powers.

Both my Tibetan teacher and my guru, Swami Sivananda, made it very clear to me to distinguish between beliefs and knowledge from personal experience. They showed me that I sometimes presented assumptions as facts. I may have some useful information, but it has to be tested to be turned into knowledge. Having a theoretical understanding and an ability to intellectualize very cleverly can deceive us into thinking that we have accomplished something.

Self-deception has to be carefully investigated. Ask yourself, Have I changed? Have I been able to get control of my mind? What have I accomplished in my attempt toward self-mastery?

You may think you are already advanced on the spiritual path if you have a moment of bliss in chanting or from doing a good deed. But that step may be very small and difficult to maintain. The spiritual path is walking the razor's edge. Whatever your achievements, don't make them bigger than they are through wishful thinking or even through the sincere desire to advance. The work that needs to be done is tremendous.

Observe how difficult it is to drop your grudges and to keep negative thoughts out of your mind. Wherever you are, you have to battle your own selfishness, your many personality aspects and your illusions. The spiritual path demands every bit of strength, energy and willpower we can muster in order to wake up from being a sleepwalker.

Discrimination and careful investigation are necessary. A believer is gullible. Something sounds good and the mind eats it up. The mind is like a ravenous beast constantly seeking new and exciting food. We are very careful about what we feed the body, checking to see if the food is good or bad. I can only assure you that it is of utmost importance to look at what you feed your mind. Give the mind the best food. Feed it the truth about yourself.

If you have grown in understanding and look at the past, you may be able to see how you have made yourself ill, how you have created your own pain, how you have created your own traps and disappointments, and how you have been lured into illusions and false beliefs by uncontrolled imagination. From the insights of the past, you can understand the present better. Then it is no miracle to anticipate the future, over which you gain some control.

Greater knowledge can best be achieved by increased concentration. The ability to keep the mental merry-go-round noises out and to become single-pointed of mind is the key to all powers. When this is understood within oneself rather than on an intellectual level, peace of mind will come.

Personal experience provides the needed evidence and encouragement to pursue knowledge of a higher nature. Insights come kindled by sincerity and devotion, humility and honesty. The Higher Self, which is a particular kind of intelligence and consciousness, will indeed try to give inspiration. If that same level of awareness with its accompanying characteristics can be maintained, the future will be a world of harmony and therefore happiness. Applying what has been learned in all situations is like a charm itself. Then awareness is not considered difficult, but rather takes on the soft gentle glow of the first glimpse of illumination. But don't listen to me, find out for yourself.

17 On Spiritual Leadership

MY PERSONAL EXPERIENCE with my teacher, Swami Sivananda, showed me that he was a man of great character and enormous compassion. I could see that from the way he treated a variety of people – taking in orphans and building a hospital for lepers. He combined this compassion with great knowledge. But he did not meet everyone's idea of what a leader is. I remember a Canadian couple visiting and saying, "He looks like a businessman," because he was wearing a coat. Naturally if it's cold in the Himalayas, you wear a coat. But their idea was that if you practise yoga, you don't need anything material and also that you should know everything. It's a very childish idea but many people start there.

What do you look for in a leader? Compassion and awareness? Or superficial things like eating habits or choice of clothes? The superficial demands very easily become grounds for criticism. From my viewpoint, the important questions are: What does the person do under certain circumstances? How are difficult situations handled?

You have to clarify to yourself what you are

looking for. If you are looking for a spiritual movie, then that's what you'll get. If you are looking for an easy, comfortable way, then you will find a teacher who offers an easy way. But if you are serious and understand that the purpose of each human life is to develop your mind and your consciousness or to find self-realization, you will look for a teacher who has something to give. In fact, you don't even need to look. You will find that teacher when you are ready. Then you must decide that you will listen.

What most people want is a good life, and then, "Oh yes, there is God, also, but that comes second." The whole thing becomes very artificial if there is no self-examination, no working on oneself. "Know thyself and be free" is as true now as it has always been, but who wants to know themselves? What I call "pseudo-gurus" never even make an attempt to wake people up, but rather lull them further into their fantasies.

People admire and follow the person who will give them what they want. From my perspective what we want to do is quite insignificant. We live to do what we ought to do, and that is furthering our own awareness. It is not even that important that we reach the ultimate self-realization, as long as we gain awareness of who we really are as individuals and understand ourselves and see our motivations and our games. That kind of work makes a person of a very different quality than somebody who just wants sugar-candy, somebody who wants something for nothing.

So you can seek a leader who fulfills your desires or someone who knows what is necessary for the evolution of consciousness.

People may start off on a genuine spiritual search and have a desire to find someone to help, but much of it may also be a fantasy. There may be an image or an idea floating around in the mind that, "If I just find somebody like that, then I will be all right, then I will know what to do." This attitude is an escape into lack of responsibility.

I remember saying to my guru, Swami Sivananda, "I will do anything you ask me, but not if it goes against my conscience." I have said the same to others: "I will ask you to do many things, but if you feel it goes against your conscience, you should tell me." Then they have to speak up. If they don't, they are probably prevented by their own image of their teacher, thinking, "Oh, I can't talk about that. I can't say that." In other words, they put the teacher outside of the realm where he or she really belongs. And again, it's their own fantasy.

I was at a symposium of spiritual leaders in San Francisco where the subject was: Do students have the right to demand that their teachers be examples or is it enough for them to pass on the teachings theoretically? The group was divided, which to me already indicated where some people were. Imagination, illusion and desire have an enormous power. People may theoretically understand this power and be quite clear about it, but when it comes to action, they fall into the trap.

The more entertainment offered and the more the leader fits the image of the seeker's dreams, the greater can be the disappointment and the ruder the awakening. Rather than looking for a teacher who fits a certain concept, whether that is a spiritual Prince Charming, a wise father figure or an always-loving mother, aspirants should instead prepare themselves to be receptive and willing to apply self-discipline. Be assured that through sincere prayer, you will find the teacher who will most benefit you.

The need to clarify our goal and purpose of life must be emphasized over and over again. No one can be relieved of this responsibility. Each of us will find what we seek; if we seek the Most High, we will find the Most High. Through our focus we attract others of like quality. Even in daily life we can see this. People who have something in common gravitate together. When our search for the Divine is single-pointed, then we will be drawn to others of Light. But this Light of knowledge doesn't just descend on us. We have to attract this Light. We have to want this Light so intensely with our total being that we become a magnet and draw this Light to ourselves.

In yoga we want to go beyond selfishness, to recognize our own divinity. We must discover this divinity within; it cannot be given by anybody. If I am told that I have a soul, what does it mean? If I fantasize about an idea that is not born of me, I may never really have contact with the soul. As Jesus said, "The Kingdom of God is within." Let us begin that journey inward, maintaining that particular state of mind that never loses sight of the ultimate reality – the Light.

18 To Teach & To Learn

BEFORE WE GO INTO the subject of how to teach yoga, we first have to ask why anyone would want to teach. What is the attraction? What is the motivation? The reasons can be varied – from imagining a certain glamour in the position, to a desire to tell others what to do, to a sincere desire to share and help. The person most qualified to teach is often the one who is least eager.

I often feel that when we express a desire to teach, we are ignorant of the enormous responsibility involved. Think about the problems we face as adults that can be traced back to those who taught us as children – our mothers, fathers and schoolteachers. Teaching a spiritual practice is not so different. The ultimate aim of the teacher must be to help people develop a higher level of awareness.

The teacher must never stop learning, realizing that students can only be taken as far as the teacher has developed himself or herself. When the process of learning stops, "teaching" is only repetition. As teachers we must continue not only to study and learn, but to apply what is learned to daily life. We also have to realize that the material we teach undergoes many changes. We often think we know Truth when we do not. We must be honest and acknowledge that we approach Truth gradually, and that the same material can be understood on many levels, depending on the development of teacher and student. A teacher must be able to see the many levels of understanding. He or she must also recognize that each student offers valuable learning experience. Those who can learn from their students have a sense of humility, which is another essential quality in a teacher.

Usually we learn by trial and error, so we must also learn to accept ourselves, including our errors. We must see ourselves as we are, not just how we want to be. If we accept only our successes, we create a false image even in our own minds. Once we can see ourselves as we are, we can decide what ideals we want to bring into our daily lives. These ideals – for example kindness, understanding, patience, a cheerful attitude – have to be firmly planted in the mind. Having established them in our minds, we have to give sufficient time and careful thought to how we will put them into practice.

By thoroughly examining ourselves, we can also deepen our compassion and understanding of others. That understanding will come across and create openness between teacher and student. As teachers we have to be careful not to judge others. What if Jesus had decided that no one was worthy enough to carry his divine message? Some of his disciples were rough and unreliable; others lacked self-confidence. We are all rather imperfect human beings. Every teacher can accept frailties in students if they also have a sense of responsibility, the right motivation and strength of commitment. When you allow people into your class, you must accept each one, exactly as they are. You may point out that you do not agree with certain actions, but you cannot condemn the individual. Being judgemental creates more damage than good. Remember that you, too, want to be accepted.

As a teacher, you also cannot be expected to be perfect. Perfection, in any case, is just a concept of the individual. Some people, however, make more effort than others to deal with their shortcomings. Some put in so much effort that their success is truly recognizable to those around them. A teacher can at least be expected to set an example to some degree. When I say to some degree, I mean that when the student sees your own struggle and goodwill, you create a good foundation for a meaningful relationship. It is important not to keep your failures hidden away like dark secrets, but rather to show your own human nature. You can give encouragement through your frankness and openness, by sharing how and what you do with your shortcomings, yet without making a display of it. To pretend means that you cannot be yourself, and therefore you cannot teach your students to become themselves.

Hatha Yoga should never be reduced to a form of gymnastics. A yoga teacher should know that the many types of yoga – Hatha, Bhakti, Jnana, Karma, Kundalini, Raja – are interlinked and interrelated. The approach and the techniques may differ, but the goal is always the same – the attainment of Cosmic Consciousness.

19 Family Life & Spiritual Work

SOMETIMES PEOPLE separate spiritual life and family life in a way that isn't realistic. You can actually accomplish a lot during the time that you are raising a family and, once your children become independent, you can focus more intensely on your spiritual aspirations. I disagree with some people who leave their young families to become *sanyasins* (renunciates). I feel it is better to become the best husband or wife, the best father or mother and friend to your children, and to use your family life to grow until you can dedicate yourself wholeheartedly to the spiritual path.

In *sanyas* there are twelve years of tapas (purification), but you can also carry out your tapas within the family – even within your physical, sexual relationship. Instead of using your partner for self-gratification or compensation, you can develop a relationship where sex is the enhancement of love and where there is a true inner giving.

So in your family life you can prepare for deeper spiritual work. Use the time to develop honesty, compassion and patience. You can also begin thinking on a deeper level – what is love, do you really love or are you only in love with the idea of loving? In Kundalini Yoga this kind of questioning is the foundation work, symbolized by the square in the first *cakra*. Ask yourself: What is consciousness? What is mind? Where do I lie? How subtle can a lie be – perhaps pretending to agree when you really don't, or acting sweetly when you are bursting with resentment? There is much you can do during the eighteen years it takes for your children to grow up. Then in your remaining years, you can become a saint! Just try it and you will see.

Family is not necessarily a hindrance to spiritual life, but it can delay your progress if you want to focus on spiritual work. Naturally if I have a husband, then I will be thinking about what he is doing – if he looks tired, or if he didn't have supper, or if he is still out somewhere in the rain. Your mind is there with your partner. It cannot be helped. Your mind is divided.

If you bring observation, awareness and humility into daily life, and quality into all your work, then it doesn't matter where you are – in an ashram, in the city, married or unmarried. Because when you have humility, observation and awareness, you know exactly how attached you are and where you need to practise non-attachment. But you have to really do it, not just leave it as an intellectual concept.

A very one-sided life is not necessarily better than any other life. I have seen someone who was considered a very holy man in India because he had practised *mauna* (silence) for ten years. But living in a cave where communication is impossible does not necessarily lead to higher development. I observed that when this man was asked one challenging question, his anger roared up. What is the use of silence and *brahmacharya* (celibacy or purity) if someone can still push your buttons and set you off? You have achieved nothing.

We are all here on Earth to learn, to grow. And therefore we have to accept the problems and difficulties in whatever choices we make. There is no ideal state, so we have to struggle through the situations in which we find ourselves. In your family you may meet the exact challenges you need. My guru told me that I was trained for my work from the day I was born. Once when I complained to him that I couldn't be anybody's spiritual mother because I didn't have a human mother who cared, he looked at me and said, "First you couldn't break loose. Then when you had a mother who set you free, you complain."

Each individual has to make their own decision about pursuing their spiritual life. Whether you are married, have children or have a career, this should not stand in the way. You can dedicate everything you do to the Most High, and bring the greatest quality possible into your life.

20 Beyond Name, Shape or Form

PRINCESS MIRA lived in the sixteenth century and meditated on the image of Lord Krishna, which is a common one in India. Krishna is a blue god shown in a bent position, playing the flute and looking very appealing. By his bent position he is saying to the worshiper, "I am lenient with your frailties." He is beautifully dressed, bedecked in jewels and decorated with peacock feathers – symbolizing that through Lord Krishna one can achieve a liberation that is much more beautiful than any jewellery the world can give. By identifying with Lord Krishna, Mira achieved what she considered *samadhi*.

Then one day, while she was meditating, Lord Krishna appeared to her and told her to go to a village some miles away where his beloved devotee, her guru, lived. He told her to study and learn from him, by meditating under his guidance.

Mira, in complete astonishment, asked Krishna, "Now that I have a constant vision of you, who could teach me anything?"

"Have you really seen me?" the Lord replied. "There is something more you have yet to see, which is the Lord in the guru."

Another way of stating Lord Krishna's truth is to say that the image a person has of the Divine is the very rival that stands in the way of truly knowing the Divine. In the same way, the ideas we have of each other are the rivals for knowing each other truly. When we identify with anyone, we identify with our image of that person, which cannot be accurate since it is coloured by our perceptions and interpretations of the mind.

Princess Mira went in search of her guru. She stayed with him until he helped her find the true state of Cosmic Consciousness, which is beyond name, shape and form. To understand what this means, try to think of yourself without your human shape and without the familiar name that has been given to you. If we want to know ourselves, it means finding out who we are beyond name and form. As long as we identify with any name or form, even a name like Krishna or Jesus or Buddha, we are still like children who identify with their parents. The little girl plays mommy and the little boy plays daddy, which is permissible for children. However, just as we expect children to grow up, the spiritual child in us is expected to grow up, too.

Even to have divine visions or to hear the voice of the Lord, as Princess Mira did, is not sufficient. You can be in heaven, but even from heaven, the gods must be reborn again. We have to go beyond heaven to that state referred to as *satcitananda*, which is pure being, pure knowledge, pure bliss.

Enlightenment is the process of detachment. We have to detach ourselves as much as possible from our ideas and images in order to proceed with our own development. It is not required that we live in pain or suffering. Neither must we renounce fulfilling our daily needs, including companionship. It is only our possessiveness and our attachments that must be relinquished. By being detached, we can truly appreciate what freedom and joy there is in life. Then life and death can be equally accepted. We do not want to develop an uncaring indifference, but a nonattachment that comes from knowing that only the physical body dies. Not even the mind dies because consciousness is energy, and energy does not die.

With what do you want to identify? That choice has to be made very carefully. We cannot think of God without the creation of an image for the mind to hold on to. It is obvious that during different stages of development, different images are but a substitution for each other. However, in the process of substitution of images, they become refined and serve as a focal point for the untrained and restless mind. Eventually the mind is trained and becomes capable of directing itself to movement of breath and image of Light.

The symbol of Light has the most subtle shape and form. The mind can use it as a transition in moving toward the formless, while expressing symbolically the most beautiful, the most perfect, the Most High. We can all meet in the Light, which will bring us together and hold us together.

Each of us has the chance to develop in the course of a lifetime according to our determination to follow our goals and our vision. But not until the mind's selfish desires are burned away will we realize the Divine. At that point, the Divine is realized not as a supreme being with shape and form, but as vibration, as energy, as power.

Either you are the master of your life and decide where you are going, or you are controlled by your emotions and the whole range of personality aspects, each with its own ego. Only you can make that decision. When you rise above selfishness and attachment to any of life's experiences, then the mystical union can take place and you will enter the state of *satcitananda*: pure being, pure knowledge, pure bliss.

Resources for the teachings of Swami Sivananda Radha

Yasodhara Ashram, yoga retreat and study centre
PO Box 9, Kootenay Bay, British Columbia
Canada V0B 1X0
(800) 661-8711
info@yasodhara.org
yasodhara.org

About the Author

SWAMI SIVANANDA RADHA (1911–1995) is regarded as one of the most profound and practical spiritual leaders of the twentieth century. Born in Germany, Swami Radha moved to Canada after World War II, and traveled to India in the 1950s to meet her spiritual teacher, Swami Sivananda. Initiated into sanyas in 1956, she then returned to Canada and dedicated her life to the yogic path.

Swami Radha founded Yasodhara Ashram in 1963, now one of the longest running spiritual centres in North America. A pioneer in the development of yoga in the West, her approach was distinguished by her unique ability to synthesize yogic teachings and western psychology.

She is a respected author of over ten books, several of which have become classics in the field of yoga, most notably *Kundalini Yoga for the West* and *Hatha Yoga: The Hidden Language*. Her published works represent a living legacy of yoga practice based on forty years of personal study and compassionate teaching.